Hemantha Dodampahala

Medical and Surgical Disorders in Pregnancy

Hemantha Dodampahala

Medical and Surgical Disorders in Pregnancy

LAP LAMBERT Academic Publishing

Impressum / Imprint

Bibliografische Information der Deutschen Nationalbibliothek: Die Deutsche Nationalbibliothek verzeichnet diese Publikation in der Deutschen Nationalbibliografie; detaillierte bibliografische Daten sind im Internet über http://dnb.d-nb.de abrufbar.

Bibliographic information published by the Deutsche Nationalbibliothek: The Deutsche Nationalbibliothek lists this publication in the Deutsche Nationalbibliografie; detailed bibliographic data are available in the Internet at http://dnb.d-nb.de.

Coverbild / Cover image: www.ingimage.com

Verlag / Publisher:
LAP LAMBERT Academic Publishing
ist ein Imprint der / is a trademark of
OmniScriptum GmbH & Co. KG
Heinrich-Böcking-Str. 6-8, 66121 Saarbrücken, Deutschland / Germany
Email: info@lap-publishing.com

Herstellung: siehe letzte Seite /
Printed at: see last page
ISBN: 978-3-659-56691-2

Medical and Surgical Disorders in Pregnancy

Professor Hemantha Dodampahala
(MBBS FRCOG MD FRCSE)
Consultant Obstetrician and Gynaecologist
Faculty of Medicine, University of Colombo, Sri Lanka

Contents

7. Other Endocrine Problems

8. Immunological disorders

9. Respiratory Diseases

10. Epilepsy

11. Diseases of Liver and the Alimentary Tract

12. Psychiatric Disorders

Medical and surgical problems in pregnancy

Pregnancy Induced Hypertension (PIH)

PIH is development of elevated blood pressure more than 140mmHg systolic or 90mmHg diastolic (which represents 3 SD values for normal distribution of blood pressure in pregnancy) generally occuring after 16-20 weeks of pregnancy in a previously normotensive mother.

Proteinuria

Proteinuria is the excretion of more than 300mg of protein per 24 hours collection in the absence of Urinary Tract Infection.Proteinuria denotes the occurrence of glomerular endotheliosis which could simultaneously occur in the other organs such as placenta causing acute on chronic placental vascular insufficiency.Similarly other major organs in the body may also suffer from similar immunological related vascular responses leading to tertiary complications of the PIH. Hence persistent proteinuria is an indication of major organ vascular endotheliosis leading to multi organ failure hence termination of pregnancy is indicated in PIH associated with gross persistent proteinuria.

The quantification of protein loss can be roughly assessed by heat coagulation of the urine.It is believed +1 protein loss is equivalent to 300 mg of daily loss and +4 protein is equivalent to 5 g of daily protein loss in urine.

Pre-eclampsia and related disorders

Pre-eclampsia (PET) is a disorder of epithelium peculiar to pregnancy which can affect every system in the body.

- ☒ It is usually characterised by hypertension, renal impairment and fluid retention, and often accompanied by proteinuria and some degree of intravascular coagulation.

- ☒ It arises as a consequence of failure of maternal adaptation to pregnancy.

- ☒ Although it usually develops in the late second trimester of pregnancy, it occurs as a result of events around implantation.

- ☒ It is totally dependent on the presence of trophoblast, hence could even occur in case of abnormal trophoblast proliferation i.e. molar pregnancy.

☒ The pathology begins in the placental bed which has been primed by genetically mediated immune responses. Hence could occur in first degree relatives. The immunity has a memory, hence second and subsequent pregnancies are at very low risk of acquiring PIH with the same partner. However changing partner for an individual counts as a first pregnancy. A pregnancy occurring many years after the first pregnancy with the same partner could also be affected due to defective immunological recognition.

Postulated mechanism for development of PET

Events in early pregnancy

☒ There is a failure of communication between the conceptus and the mother, possibly due to genetically mediated abnormal immunology operating at the level of the vascular endothelium of the placenta.

☒ The mother fails (either totally or partially) to adapt physiologically.

☒ Among the consequences may be:

— trophoblast fails to invade maternal spiral arterioles ---the predominance of vasodilatory PGI2 and NO in the endothelium does not occur, so vessels remain responsive to vasoconstrictors

— maternal plasma volume fails to expand

— placental bed fails to become a 'low-pressure supply system'.

— placental bed vasculature become increasingly sensitive to circulating vasoconstrictors in the maternal plasma

Prodromal phase
Placental effects (primary pathology).
☒ The placenta is perfused under high pressure

☒ Local endothelial damage causes aggregation of platelets, fibrin and lipid-laden macrophages ('acute atherosis') and micro-thrombi formation

☒ Spiral arterioles become totally or partially occluded

☒ Placental perfusion to the fetus decreases

☒ Placental size is reduced

☒ Endothelial damage begins to extend throughout the maternal vascular tree.

Fetal growth restriction.

Maternal effects
☒ Vascular resistance (VR) remains high, possibly due to poor vascular response and increased response to circulating vasoconstrictors.

☒ Cardiac output (CO) is increased

☒ The physiological fall in blood pressure (VR x CO) does not occur

☒ At a variable point thereafter, blood pressure begins to rise.

Clinical phase

This classically occurs in the late second and the third trimester.
☒ Placental infarction and sometimes, abruption may occur.

☒ Pre-eclampsia is the commonest cause of:

— IUGR in non-malformed infants

— elective pre-term delivery.

☒ Increased perinatal mortality:

— in severe disease of early onset (10- to 15-fold)

— when eclampsia occurs.

☒ Generalised maternal endothelial damage affects every system in the body with the following maternal effects.

Maternal clinical aspects of PET

The syndrome affects each woman differently. Not all aspects are apparent in each case. Every system can be affected, to a variable and sometimes severe degree.

Cardiovascular and pulmonary effects

☒ Hypertension is the commonest manifestation.

☒ Peripheral oedema occurs due to 'leaky' endothelium.

☒ Severe pre-eclampsia is a high cardiac output state with inappropriately high systemic vascular resistance. Left ventricular function is hyperdynamic: cardiac failure may supervene in the most severe cases.

- ☒ Pulmonary oedema may arise due to an imbalance between a reduced colloid osmotic pressure and the pulmonary capillary wedge pressure. It can also be precipitated by intravenous fluid overload during treatment without proper monitoring.

- ☒ Acute respiratory distress syndrome (ARDS), CVA and thromboembolism are the leading causes of death among the complicated PIH patients.

The kidney

- ☒ Glomerular endothelial cells swell, blocking the capillaries. (This 'glomerular endotheliosis' is characteristic but not pathognomonic.)

- ☒ Impairment of renal function may result in a rise in plasma uric acid (an early feature), urea and creatinine. Proteinuria develops: pre-eclampsia is the commonest cause of heavy proteinuria in pregnancy.

The liver

Liver involvement must be considered in all cases of severe pre-eclampsia.
- ☒ Hepato-cellular (periportal liver cell necrosis) damage can occur due to fibrin deposits in the sinusoids.
- ☒ Epigastric pain (due to hepatic oedema and distension of the liver capsule) and vomiting are associated with fulminating pre-eclampsia.

- ☒ In some cases, jaundice and severe liver damage can follow, often out of proportion to other signs and symptoms.

- ☒ The potentially dangerous HELLP syndrome (Haemolysis, Elevated Liver enzymes, and Low Platelets) must be considered in severe cases. The HELLP syndrome is classified by the Mississippi classification based on the number of platelets.

- ☒ Subcapsular haemorrhages and even liver rupture may occur.

Coagulation

- ☒ Increasingly generalised endothelial damage commonly causes slight intravascular coagulation, shown by increased platelet turnover and a fall in platelet count (which can be severe in some cases).

- ☒ Disseminated intravascular coagulation (DIC) with altered factor VIII antigen ratios is a rare but serious end point in some cases. This characterized by increased bleeding time, clotting time, increased venous clot retraction time and elevated D-dimer levels and low platelet levels in the serum.

- ☒ Haemolysis can occur due to fibrinogen-associated red cell aggregation.

Central nervous system

- ☒ Among the signs of CNS involvement are atypical headache, hyperreflexia, visual disturbances and ankle clonus.

- ☒ Vasoconstriction of cerebral vessels occurs (probably as a protective mechanism against severe hypertension).

- ☒ At a mean arterial pressure of about 130-150 mmHg this mechanism begins to fail, and small vessel walls-are damaged and disrupted.

- ☒ This can lead to cerebral oedema, haemorrhages and infarcts—all associated with eclampsia, a major cause of maternal death.

Maternal mortality and pre-eclampsia/eclampsia

'Hypertensive disorders of pregnancy' were the second commonest cause, after hemorrhagic deaths of maternal death in the developing countries. The thromboembolism is still the leading cause of maternal deaths in developed countries.

Predisposing factors for Pregnancy Induced Hypertention

- ☒ *Primigravidity.* The incidence of severe (proteinuric) pre-eclampsia in a first pregnancy is around 6%.The general incidence of all types of PIH may be increased up 10% in urban Sri Lankan population.

- — It occurs in about 2% of all second pregnancies, rising to 12% if severe pre-eclampsia (with IUGR) was present in the first, and falling to 0.7% if the first was a singleton, normotensive pregnancy

- — Pregnancy by a new partner may increase the risk to that of a first pregnancy

- — The protection offered by an early spontaneous or induced abortion with regard to subsequent development of hypertension need further studies.

- ☒ *Genetic.* It is either due to a dominant gene with varying penetrance or due to a 'multifactorial' inheritance. Risk is outlined in the information box.

	Excess risk in women being considered
Mother	x (4-5)
Sister	x (3-4)
Grandmother	x (2-3)

- It is also more common when there is a strong family history of hypertension, other cardiovascular disorders or auto-immune disease

- There is no significant racial preponderance.

☒ *Medical.* Among the predisposing factors are pre-existing hypertension, diabetes mellitus, protein S deficiency, activated protein C resistance, anti-cardiolipin antibodies, SLE and renal disorders.

☒ *Socioeconomic.* The incidence increases as socioeconomic status deteriorates (associated with poor maternal nutrition). The incidence is lower in women who smoke, but the fetal outlook is poor in smokers who develop pre-eclampsia. Elderly, obese professionals have a higher risk of developing PIH.

☒ *Obstetric.* Multiple pregnancy and hydatidiform mole are associated with very early and severe pre-eclampsia. It also may occur when hydrops fetalis (Rhesus and non-Rhesus) is present.

Prevention of pre-eclampsia

Low-dose aspirin. suppresses production of thromboxane A2 by platelets in vitro without significantly affecting prostacyclin.
- However, the results of published trials do not support routine prophylactic or therapeutic use in women judged to be beneficial for recurrent PIH and IUGR.

- There may be a small additional risk of ante- or postpartum haemorrhage.

- The only women in whom it may be justified are those with a previous history of eclampsia

Calcium. Randomised controlled trials (RCTs) have, so far, been too small to provide reliable information but calcium supplementation (2 g/day) during pregnancy may reduce the risk of hypertension, pre-eclampsia and pre-term delivery. Larger trials are necessary.
Fish oils. It has been suggested their use during pregnancy is associated with a fall in incidence of severe pre-eclampsia and pre- term delivery. No recommendations can yet be made from available trials.

Management of pre-eclampsia

The principles are:
- ☒ Early recognition of the symptomless syndrome

- ☒ Awareness of serious nature of the condition in its severe form without over-reacting to mild disease

- ☒ Agreed guidelines for admission to hospital, investigation, and use of anti hypertensive and anticonvulsant therapy

- ☒ Well-timed delivery to pre-empt serious maternal or fetal complications

- ☒ Correct multi-disciplinary management at an ICU setting in terms of intra-vascular fluid management, control of blood pressure and fits, seizure prophylaxis and timely delivery.

- ☒ Postnatal follow-up and counselling for future pregnancies.

Clinical observation and investigation

Examination (over and above routine):
- ☒ Palpation of the femoral pulses (to exclude coarctation of aorta)

- ☒ Look for hyperreflexia and ankle clonus

- ☒ Check optic fundi for silver wiring, arterio-venous nipping, exudates and haemorrhage.

Laboratory investigation
- ☒ Proteinuria. If present also check urine microscopy and culture to exclude urinary infection.

- ☒ Serum uric acid levels increase early in pre-eclampsia. Levels >350 umol/L are abnormal in pregnancy but gradually increasing levels are more significant.

- ☒ Serum urea and creatinine. Rising levels are significant but not such sensitive indicators of pre-eclampsia as uric acid. The upper limits of normal in pregnancy are 5 mmol/L for serum urea and 100 umol/L for creatinine, but trends are even more important than specific levels.

- ☒ Platelet count gradually falls with the rise of D-dimer if disseminated intravascular coagulation is occurring.

- ☒ Liver function—this should be checked once persistent proteinuria is present, or if platelet count is significantly reduced. It can be detected by elevation of liver enzymes (not alkaline phosphatase, which is normally raised because it is produced by the placenta).

☒ Coagulation studies should be carried out if platelet count is reduced, and in severe disease.

☒ Tests of fetal growth and well-being.

☒ Each of these tests should be repeated as often as is clinically necessary.

Management of mild (non-proteinuric) pre-eclampsia
The principles are:

☒ Uncomplicated hypertension is suitable for careful supervision by the primary health care team (MOH, PHNS, FHW)

☒ The use of sedatives or tranquillisers are contraindicated

☒ Anti hypertensive therapy is not indicated

☒ Admission to hospital is indicated when:

— SBP is 160 and/or DBP 100 mmHg or greater

— proteinuria is detected in a clean (i.e. mid-stream) urine sample in the absence of a urinary infection

— the patient is symptomatic with e.g. visual disturbances, unusual headache, epigastric pain, or vomiting (URGENT!)

— there is clinical evidence of intrauterine growth retardation — tests of fetal welfare have deteriorated

— a previous bad obstetric history suggests that closer surveillance would be worthwhile.

— Any reduction in fetal movements, tightening of the abdomen with pain and bleeding PV indicative of an abruption.

Management of severe hypertension

☒ The maternal risks of cerebrovascular accident and of left ventricular or renal failure begin to increase significantly when hypertension is severe.

☒ Correct multi-disciplinary management at an ICU setting in terms of intra-vascular fluid management, control of blood pressure and fits, seizure prophylaxis and timely delivery.

☒ The choice has then to be made between delivery and anti-hypertensive therapy.

☒ Among the factors to be considered are:

- gestational age—it is seldom justified to commence long-term oral therapy from 34 weeks
- the severity of other signs and symptoms
- availability of intensive neonatal care facilities.

☒ Treatment neither influences the progression of underlying pre-eclampsia nor improves fetal outcome. It helps to protect the mother from CVA and Cardiac Failure and enables many pregnancies to continue that otherwise would be ended because of maternal risk.

Control of acute-severe hypertension

☒ There is no consensus on the optimum acute treatment.

☒ The important objective is to reduce the blood pressure to safe levels (but not too low!).

☒ *Parenteral hydralazine* is used most commonly but oral nifedipine should be considered.

Longer-term control of severe hypertension

☒ There is still insufficient trial evidence to determine whether the benefits outweigh any disadvantages.

☒ If it is to be used, the suggested indications are:

- DBP >_100 mmHg
- pregnancy <_34 weeks
- Fetal and maternal state otherwise good.

☒ *Methyldopa* remains the drug of first choice.

☒ The combined α and β blocking agent labetalol is commonly used.

☒ The potent vasodilator and calcium channel blocker nifedipine is a useful second-line treatment. Its major drawback is severe headache.

☒ Angiotensin-converting enzyme (ACE) inhibitors have deleterious fetal effects and their use is not recommended. If a woman with chronic hypertension becomes pregnant on an ACE inhibitor, change to another anti-hypertensive agent is advised.

Diuretics

Review of trials does not allow reliable-conclusions to be reached. Their use has been discouraged in pre-eclampsia because they further reduce circulating blood volume.

Timing of delivery

Hypertension occurring in and around the term needs immediate delivery
The most common grounds for delivery are:
— progressive fetal compromise (i.e. when the baby is safer delivered)

— unacceptable risk to maternal health, e.g. uncontrollable BP, impending renal failure or heart failure, HELLP syndrome, DIC, eclampsia (see below).

☒ The mode of delivery (caesarean section versus vaginal) depends on:

— the seriousness of the situation

— the gestational age

— the favorability and Bishop's score of the cervix

— the degree of fetal/maternal compromise.

☒ Epidural analgesia is the method of choice for labour (as long as a coagulation defect has been excluded).

☒ Appropriate facilities for the care of the newborn infant must be available.

Fluid balance and plasma volume expansion

☒ Restriction of iv. fluids to less than 1 litre following delivery of women with severe pre-eclampsia reduces the risk of pulmonary oedema without affecting renal function.

☒ Diuretics are contraindicated because they aggravate hypovolaemia and can precipitate renal failure.

☒ Plasma volume expansion accompanied by vasodilator drugs (e.g. hydralazine) may have a role in some severe cases with the following provisos:

— it must be used only in high-dependency units where invasive monitoring (e.g. to measure pulmonary capillary wedge pressure— PCWP) is available

— Usually 85ml/h fluid supplement is optimal. Sometimes 35-50ml plus the previous hours urine output is appropriate.

— Blind therapy is very dangerous and can lead to pulmonary oedema, ARDS and death.

☒ Central venous pressure (CVP) monitoring may not be adequate. Measurement of PCWP may be required to prevent the occurrence of ARDS.

Eclampsia

☒ Defined as the occurrence of one or more generalized tonic-clonic convulsions in association with the syndrome of pre-eclampsia.

☒ The timing of fits follows: antepartum 38%; intrapartum 18%; postpartum 44%.

☒ Postpartum fits usually occur within 24 hours of delivery, but rarely occur up to 3 weeks later.

☒ Eclampsia is still a major contributor to maternal mortality.

☒ In addition to severe hypertension and proteinuria (which may not occur!), among the other symptoms and signs suggesting impending eclampsia are:

— unusual headache—persistent, severe, generalised (but may be occipital or frontal)

— visual disturbance—e.g. blurring, flashes or spots, photophobia

— restlessness, agitation

— epigastric pain, nausea and vomiting

— hyperreflexia and clonus

— retinal oedema, haemorrhages and even papilloedema.

Management

☒ Prevention of convulsions: intravenous and/or intramuscular magnesium sulphate has been used for many years in the developed countries for the prevention (and treatment) of eclampsia. There is some trial evidence suggesting benefit to both mother and baby.

☒ Control of convulsions: the Collaborative Eclampsia Trial has demonstrated clearly that magnesium sulphate is the drug of choice for treatment of eclampsia. It reduces neuromuscular irritability by reducing the calcium mediated vasospasm and causes lowering of the cerebral threshold. The suggested regimes are either:

— loading dose of 4 g iv or deep intramuscular(buttocks). over 5 minutes

or

— i.v. infusion of 1 g/h for 24 h

— further 2-4 g given i.v. over 5 min if convulsions recur.

Treatment is monitored clinically by checking respiratory rate (>16/min); urine output (>25 ml/h); and the continuing presence of knee jerks. Serum measurement of magnesium levels is not required. If the patient has a low urine output, half of the above mentioned doses are recommended.

☒ Control of hypertension

☒ General management

— Patency of the airway must be maintained and oxygen given as necessary

— A urinary catheter should be inserted to monitor urine output

— Check for disorders of electrolyte balance and disseminated intravascular coagulation.

— Use of dexamethasone to mature the fetal lungs i.m. 12.5mg, 2 doses 12 hours apart.

☒ *Delivery of the infant.* Caesarean section is the method of choice but only when the eclampsia is under control. If eclampsia supervenes

when the patient is well advanced in labour, vaginal delivery may be possible.

☒ **NSAIDs must be avoided for post-operative analgesia because of the risk of renal failure when used in the presence of severe pre-eclampsia!**

Long-term outlook

☒ It has for long been thought that severely pre-eclamptic/ eclamptic primigravidae are not at increased risk of developing chronic hypertension (given that there is not pre-existing hypertension). There is some evidence that this may not be the case.

☒ Patients with severe early-onset pre-eclampsia should be screened for protein S and protein C deficiency, activated protein C resistance, anti-cardiolipin antibodies, hyperhomocystinaemia and chronic hypertension because of their increased prevalence in such women.

Chronic hypertensive disorders and renal hypertension

Definitions

Hypertension—two consecutive measurements of diastolic blood pressure (DBP) ~90 mmHg 4 or more hours apart or one measurement ≥110 mm Hg. These patients have higher booking blood pressure which settles to normotensive values in most pregnancies due to pregnancy vascular changes. However 25-40% of patients may develop superimposed PIH.

☒ The DBP is traditionally taken at the 'point of muffling' (Korotkoff phase IV) in women lying on their side with a 15-30° tilt.

☒ The use of systolic blood pressure (SBP) or the calculation of mean arterial pressure does not add to the prognostic significance and is more complicated.

☒ A DBP of 90 mmHg corresponds to the point at which the perinatal mortality rate begins to rise in population studies, and is approximately the mean +3 SD in mid-pregnancy, the mean +2 SD from 34 to 37 weeks, and the mean +1 SD at term. The significance of the same level of hypertension, therefore, varies with the stage in pregnancy at which it is recorded.

Severe hypertension—a DBP >120 mmHg on one occasion or a DBP ≥110 mmHg on two consecutive occasions 4 or more hours apart.

Chronic (pre-existing) hypertension
Possible causes are:

☒ Essential hypertension—outlook is good in this condition but pre-eclampsia may supervene.

☒ Coarctation of the aorta

☒ Renal hypertension

☒ Phaeochromocytoma

☒ Auto-immune connective tissue disorders

☒ Some drugs, e.g. corticosteroids, MAO (monoamine oxidase) inhibitors.

Urinary tract infections

Asymptomatic bacteriuria

Definition: Cultured urine contains >100 000 organisms/ml.
☒ Asymptomatic bacteriuria occurs in about 5% of pregnancies.

☒ Escherichia coli (E. coli) is the infecting organism in 90% of cases.

☒ Pregnancy does not predispose to it but it progresses to acute
pyelonephritis in a greater proportion (25-40%) of pregnant women.

☒ Routine culture of a mid-stream urine (MSU) should be performed at
booking because:

— detection and treatment prevents at least two thirds of the cases of
acute pyelonephritis

— detection and successful treatment prevents preterm labour and
resultant perinatal morbidity and mortallity.This is very important
with previous preterm labour who suffered with symptomatic and
asymptomatic bacteriuria

— maternal anaemia and IUGR may be more common in untreated
cases.

☒ Recurrent bacteriuria is common.

Acute pyelonephritis

☒ This usually presents as a febrile illness with loin pain and vomiting.

☒ It needs to be differentiated from other causes of an acute abdomen.

☒ It is associated with pre-term labour, IUGR and IUD.

☒ Blood cultures should be taken in severe cases. E. coli is the commonest
infecting organism.

☒ Treatment with appropriate antibiotic should begin while urine culture and
sensitivity results are awaited. It should continue in full therapeutic
doses for 3-6 weeks. Thereafter urine culture should be performed from
each antenatal visit.

☒ If it recurs consider maintenance antibacterial therapy for the remainder of
pregnancy and for 2 weeks postpartum.

Chronic renal disease

- Pregnancy perse does not usually adversely affect most renal diseases, with the possible exception of membrano-proliferative glomerulonephritis and lupus nephropathy. Chronic renal disease with high creatinine carries high peri-natal mortality rate. Eg. Serum creatinine more than 2mg/dl carries over 50% pregnancy loses.

- The increased risk of urinary infection in pregnancy can lead to exacerbation of chronic pyelonephritis.

- The outcome of pregnancy is proportional to the severity of renal impairment rather than specific diseases.

Pre-pregnancy counselling

- Pregnancy is not advisable in women whose plasma creatinine levels are 2mg/dl and whose DBP is ~90 mmHg. Most women with severe renal impairment are amenorrhoeic and infertile.If the patient is on ACE Inhibitors consider Methyldopa or slow acting Nifedipine as ACE Inhibitors may cause feral renal failure and severe oligohydroamnios.

- Among the renal diseases seen in pregnancy are:

  — chronic pyelonephritis—good prognosis if renal function adequate and normotensive

  — chronic glomerulonephritis—patients more liable to develop superadded pre-eclampsia

  — polycystic kidneys—prognosis depends on renal function and level of Blood Pressure

  — auto-immune connective tissue disease nephropathy

  — diabetic nephropathy

- Regular antenatal assessment should be carried out with the help of nephrologist and a physician.The disease requires monitoring of

  — maternal blood pressure, renal function and urine cultures

  — fetal growth and well-being

NEPHROTIC SYNDROME

Heavy proteinuria (>3.5 g/24 h), with hypoalbuminaemia and gross generalised oedema.

☒ The commonest cause in late pregnancy is pre-eclampsia.

☒ If it occurs before 32 weeks' gestation a high-protein diet can be given and salt-free albumin infusions considered after seeking advice from a nephrologist.

☒ Steroids should not be given unless a biopsy-proven diagnosis suggests that they would be beneficial (e.g. membranoproliferative glomerulonephritis).

☒ Diuretics are contraindicated.

Renal and ureteric calculi

If this diagnosis is suspected, intravenous urography is indicated if two of the following are present:

☒ Microscopic haematuria

☒ Recurrent symptoms referable to urinary tract

☒ Sterile urine culture when symptoms suggest pyelonephritis.

Management is initially conservative, with hydration, antibiotics and analgesia. Surgery is rarely necessary.

Renal allografts and pregnancy

☒ Chronic haemodialysis is associated with infertility, and successful pregnancy is uncommon in women receiving this treatment.

☒ Renal transplantation restores fertility in proportion to reproductive age and allograft function.

Pre-pregnancy counselling

☒ The following criteria are guides to the timing of pregnancy:

— at least 18 months since transplant

— renal function stable, with no proteinuria and plasma creatinine ≤200 umol/L

— normotensive (or nearly so)

— no evidence of graft rejection

— immunosuppressive therapy at maintenance levels and immunosuppression with azathioprine is safe during the pregnancy

- Antenatal care should be hospital-based in a joint clinic involving obstetrician and nephrologist.

- In addition to routine, maternal assessment should include screening for anaemia, any infection, and superadded pre-eclampsia.

- Graft rejection is no more or less common. Renal ultrasonography may be helpful in its detection. Immunosuppressive therapy should be maintained. The effects of cyclosporin therapy in pregnancy need to be evaluated for its teratogenic effect,However azathioprine is safe during the pregnancy.

- Vaginal delivery should be aimed for. Caesarean section is indicated for obstetric reasons only.

- Fetal outcome is satisfactory in the absence of pre-term labour (elective and spontaneous) and IUGR. Congenital malformations are not more common. Neonates may be more prone to viral or other infections. The risk of congenital abnormality is not increased.

There is disagreement as to whether breast-feeding is safe as long as mother in not on teratogenic immune suppressants. Postpartum contraception poses a problem. On balance, a low- dose combined pill,Intrauterine contraceptive device(Cu T 380),barrier methods may be best as long as surveillance is frequent.

Anaemia

- The haemoglobin (Hb) concentration falls during pregnancy (but not normally below 10g/dl) because the physiological increase in plasma volume outstrips that of the red cell mass.

- The average requirement for iron is about 4 mg/day, increasing as the pregnancy progresses. Although the normal diet contains up to 25 mg/day of iron only about 10% of this is absorbed. Iron stores fall, therefore, during pregnancy. The first effect is a fall in serum ferritin to around 6 ug/L by 28 weeks. Hb does not fall, and microcytic erythrocytes do not appear for several weeks after the stores are exhausted.

- At present trial data do not recommend routine supplementation with iron and folate of all pregnant women in well-nourished communities. However we come across a mixed population in Sri Lanka (i.e. majority lower marginal or low). Hence routine supplementation is proven to be beneficial and cost effective.

Iron deficiency

1) The blood film is hypochromic and microcytic.

2) Mean corpuscular haemoglobin (MCH) is decreased.

3) Serum ferritin levels are low (<15 µg/L).

4) Iron-binding capacity is increased.

Treatment

In ward acute treatment of anaemia is indicated in any high risk pregnancy, especially associated with conditions that will predispose to antepartum or postpartum haemorrhage. Eg. Placenta preavia, twin pregnancy, as these patients have a higher chance of antepartum and postpartum haemorrhage.

- ☒ Increase dietary sources of iron (e.g. meat, fish, eggs,green leafy vegetables and spinach) and supplement with oral iron. If gastrointestinal intolerance to iron occurs, change to a chelated or delayed-release preparation. Parenteral iron therapy is a good alternative during early pregnancy which reduces the incidence of blood transfusion.

- ☒ Blood transfusion is necessary in patients who are proven to be anaemic with a risk of subsequent postpartum haemorrhage.

- ☒ An underlying folate deficiency may be unmasked by treatment, hence folate supplementation 5mg per day is recommended.

Folate deficiency

Blood film is normochromic and macrocytic. Red cells may be nucleated and contain Howell—Jolly nuclear inclusion bodies.
- ☒ Check serum folate and B12 (red cell folate is low in both folate and B12 deficiency and is therefore not so helpful. Folate deficiency is associated with an increased risk of neural tube defects, placental abruption, occurrence of PIH and megaloblastic anaemia.

Treatment

Increase dietary sources of folate (as for iron). Give 5-15 mg folic acid orally daily.In patients suffering from Pernicious anaemia Vitamin B12 is given parenterally.

Vitamin B12 deficiency

- ☒ Vitamin B12 deficiency is rare in pregnancy, with a higher incidence in strict vegetarians. Blood film is megaloblastic.

- ☒ Treatment is with intramuscular vitamin B12. A daily folate supplement of 300 ug will not mask vitamin B12 deficiency.

Sickle cell disease

This is an autosomal recessive disorder characterised by denaturation of the haemoglobin at low partial pressures of oxygen leading to vascular obstruction, DVT, placental infarction and IUD.

- ☒ Major problem is Hb S/S, with Hb S/C and Hb S/Thal being less common

- ☒ Perinatal loss and IUGR are common.

Sickling crises- Hb A and its abnormal variants function similarly when well-oxygenated but the latter polymerise when deoxygenated. The red cells become sickle-shaped and occlude vessels, causing widespread vascular damage, severe pain and haemolytic anaemia.

Prevention Folate supplements and oral bicarbonate (to increase the pH of the urine); blood transfusion (3-4 units) at 6-week intervals; prompt treatment of infection.

Sickle cell trait (Hb A/S)
This is usually benign, but sickling cases occur under extreme hypoxia. The Hb level tends to be lower than average. It may predispose to pyelonephritis.

Management of severe anaemia in pregnancy
- ☒ If Hb is <6.0 g/dl then consider exchange transfusion or plasmaphoresis.

- ☒ If Hb is between 6.0 and 8.0 g/dl then transfuse slowly with 3-5 units of packed cells. Use intravenous frusemide 20 mg to prevent circulatory overload.

Cardiac disease

The haemodynamic changes which occur during pregnancy impose an increased burden on the mother's heart. This causes no problems for healthy women but may do so in women with cardiac disease.

Rheumatic heart disease (RHD)

- ☒ The incidence of RHD has decreased dramatically over the past 25 years in most developed countries.

- ☒ Mitral stenosis is still the commonest and most important problem.

- ☒ Pregnancy has no permanent deleterious effect on RHD.

Congenital heart deffects (CHD)

☒ An increasing number of women with CHD are reaching childbearing age as a result of improved medical and surgical management.

☒ Most women with acyanotic CHD tolerate pregnancy well (except those with severe aortic stenosis and coarctation of the aorta). The cardiac disease become serious when there is fixed output failure due to aortic,pulmonary or mitral stenosis or pulmonary hypertension.

☒ Patients with uncorrected CHD, pulmonary hypertension (either primary or as part of Eisenmenger's syndrome) do badly, and maternal death can occur suddenly. Progression to pulmonary hypertension causes serious output failure.

Other cardiac lesions

☒ Tachyarrhythmias can be managed on temporary or pacemaker.There is a limited choice for medical management

☒ Myocardial infarction—a rare complication of pregnancy; risk factors include smoking, hypertension, diabetes mellitus and familial hypercholesterolaemia.

☒ Severe cardiac failure and arrest --immediate termination of the pregnancy is indicated to relieve the heart and facilitate the resuscitation in Cardiac arrest.

Pre-conception counselling

This is important for women with known heart disease because:

☒ Treatment can be made optimal

☒ A specific plan can be prepared for pregnancy

☒ Surgery can be advised in those women in whom pregnancy would add a severe but correctable burden, e.g. tight mitral stenosis

☒ Advice can be given to those women at high risk during pregnancy, e.g. Marfan's syndrome, inoperable cyanotic heart disease, primary pulmonary hypertension, Eisenmenger's syndrome; pregnancy may be best avoided in these conditions.

Antenatal management

Termination of pregnancy is not medically indicated, except when pulmonary hypertension is severe.

- ☒ Arrange regular antenatal visits to obstetrician and cardiologist.

- ☒ Ensure adequate rest.

- ☒ Strongly advise against smoking.

- ☒ Prevent anaemia.

- ☒ Treat respiratory infection promptly.

- ☒ Cover dental work with antibiotics.

- ☒ Be watchful for incipient pulmonary congestion and arrhythmias.

Management of labour

- ☒ Aim for vaginal delivery at term. Induction of labour is necessary only for obstetric reasons. Vaginal prostaglandins are the method of choice because early amniotomy may increase the risk of infection.

- ☒ When patient starts labour with good cardiac reserve the risk of heart failure is low.

- ☒ Cover labour with antibiotics.

- ☒ Control any infusion of parenteral fluids very strictly.

- ☒ Provide adequate analgesia—epidural anaesthesia is safe in experienced hands as long as hypotension is avoided; it is contraindicated in hypertrophic obstructive cardiomyopathy (HOLM) (see below) and Eisenmenger's syndrome.

- ☒ Avoid aortocaval compression.

- ☒ Shorten the second stage by use of 'lift-out' forceps or vacuum extractor (without raising legs into lithotomy position if possible).

- ☒ Ergometrine is avoided.

- ☒ Do not attempt caesarean section in the presence of heart failure.

- ☒ Have oxygen and relevant drugs immediately available.

- ☒ Avoid β-sympathomimetic drugs in women with pre-existing heart disease.

Specific problems
Cardiac failure

- ☒ The principles of diagnosis and treatment are the same as in the non-pregnant patient.
- ☒ It can occur even in young asymptomatic women with cardiac disease at any stage of pregnancy.

☒ Sudden cardiac decompensation is more likely to occur shortly after delivery.

Acute pulmonary oedema

A medical emergency which demands immediate attention.

Management
☒ Nurse in semi-recumbent position, give oxygen and keep airways clear.

☒ Give intravenous morphine, aminophylline, frusemide and digoxin (if not previously digitalised). In labour the fetus must take second place until the situation is under control.

Tachyarrhythmias

Atrial fibrillation is a medical emergency requiring bed rest in hospital and digitalisation. The advice of a cardiologist must always be sought. Anticoagulation may also be indicated.

Atrial tachycardia can precipitate heart failure rapidly. It often responds to carotid sinus pressure.

Cardiac surgery and pregnancy
Cardiac surgery if required is usually performed in second trimester.
☒ Anticoagulant therapy must be maintained and carefully controlled in women who have had previous cardiac surgery.

☒ Warfarin is the drug of choice here even in the first trimester. Intravenous heparin should be substituted 2-3 weeks before anticipated time of delivery.

☒ Mitral valvotomy-PTMC (Percutaneous Trans Mitral Commissurotomy may be indicated during pregnancy in pure severe mitral stenosis if pulmonary congestion develops, or if there is no prompt response to medical therapy.

Hypertrophic obstructive cardiomyopathy (HOCM)
☒ Most women with HOCM tolerate pregnancy and vaginal delivery well. This depends, however, on the severity of the left ventricular outflow tract obstruction.

☒ It is important to avoid:
— digoxin therapy
— β-sympathomimetic drugs—some of the deaths associated with their use have been in women with undiagnosed cardiomyopathy
— aortocaval compression—e.g. the left lateral position should be used for delivery.

☒ Caesarean section should be reserved for obstetric indications.

Diabetes mellitus (DM)

This could be divided into
1) Gestational Diabetes Mellitus

2) Pre-gestational Diabetes Mellitus (Established Diabetes Mellitus)

Definition

Fasting venous plasma glucose concentration ≥8.0 mmol/L and ≥11.0 mmol/L 2 hours after a 75 g oral glucose load; or one of these plus symptoms and signs (polydipsia, polyuria, weight loss).

Impaired glucose tolerance (IGT) is present if the fasting level is <8.0 mmol/L but rises to 8.0-10.9 mmol/L 2 hours after 75 g oral glucose load.

Antenatal screening

IGT/DM must be suspected in all women with:
☒ Significant glycosuria on two occasions antenatally or in a single fasting urine sample

☒ Mother, father or siblings with diabetes

☒ Previous babies >90th percentile for gestational age and sex

☒ Diabetes in a previous pregnancy

☒ Previous unexpected perinatal death

☒ Polyhydramnios

☒ Maternal obesity (>20% above ideal weight).

Routine antenatal screening has been recommended because:
☒ About 30% of gestational diabetes patients have none of the above risk features

☒ Not all women with IGT or even diabetes have persistent glycosuria

☒ Glycosuria can be found in the urine of up to 50% of all pregnant women at some time.

Selective or comprehensive screening can be undertaken by:

☒ Estimation of blood glucose concentrations fasting and 2 hours after a 50 g glucose load. An oral 75 g glucose tolerance test (GTT) is indicated if fasting and/or the 2-hour levels exceed 5 and 7 mmol/L respectively.

Risks associated with diabetes

All risks are increased by poor control of diabetes (especially if keto-acidosis develops) and by inadequate obstetric supervision.

☒ Maternal—retinopathy, nephropathy and neuropathy may be worsened

☒ Congenital malformations—there is a slight general increase in malformations related to hyperglycaemia during organogenesis, especially craniospinal and cardiac defects; sacral agenesis is a rare anomaly specifically associated with diabetes.The risk of malformation proportionate to the abnormality of glycemia as detected with HbA1C.

☒ Obstetric complications—e.g. polyhydramnios, pre-term labour, pre-eclampsia

☒ Infections—urinary,candidal and other infections

☒ Sudden unexpected fetal death (SUFD)—increased risk during the last 4-6 weeks of pregnancy

☒ Difficult delivery—because of excess fetal growth (macrosomia) and shoulder dystocia,Increased risk of instrumental delivery and caesarean section

☒ Neonatal problems—birth trauma, hyaline membrane disease, hypoglycaemia, hypomagnesaemia, hypocalcaemia, jaundice.

☒ Macrosomia has been reported in up to 30% of seemingly well-controlled diabetics.

Management

Pre-pregnancy counselling allows:

☒ General advice, e.g. about tight diabetic control (particularly around conception and in the early weeks of pregnancy)

☒ Planning for pregnancy (including early booking for antenatal care)

- ☒ Review of diet

- ☒ Examination of optic fundi/ peripheral vessels and look for PVD and blood pressure.

- ☒ Establishment of good blood glucose control.

Antenatal care for pre-existing diabetics should be jointly between obstetrician and physician. For optimal diabetic control:

- ☒ Organise high-fibre diet with correct calorific intake and CHO content

- ☒ Carry out blood glucose profiles two or three times/week at home using filter-paper strips or a reflectance meter. Tests are carried out before and 2 hours after each meal and last thing at night. Pre- and post-prandial levels of <5.0 and <7.0 mmol/L respectively are ideal

- ☒ Regular urinalysis (mainly to check on carbohydrate loss)

- ☒ Regular glycosylated haemoglobin or fructosamine estimations (mainly to provide retrospective information on the validity of home glucose monitoring)

- ☒ Insulin treatment is best using combined soluble and intermediate-acting insulins morning and evening or intermittent soluble insulin with each meal (three times a day) and an intermediate acting insulin in the evening. Human or highly purified porcine insulins reduce the risk of developing antibodies (which can cross the placenta)

- ☒ Maternal health is also monitored carefully, paying particular attention to weight, optic fundi, blood pressure, and renal function

- ☒ Fetal welfare should be monitored carefully:

  - — Carry out baseline scans to confirm gestational age and, at 20 weeks', to exclude major anomalies (especially cranio-spinal and cardiac defects)

  - — Continue with serial scans for reduced and, particularly, excess fetal growth

  - — Assess fetal well-being regularly from 28 weeks

  - — If macrosomia arises check ultrasound scans for fetal cardiac enlargement.

Admission to hospital is indicated if:

- ☒ Good glucose control cannot be achieved as an outpatient

- ☒ Severe hypertension or pre-eclampsia develop

- ☒ Weight gain is excessive
- ☒ Renal function deteriorates
- ☒ Fetal well-being causes concern.

Gestational diabetes

- ☒ If IGT is discovered during pregnancy, carry out blood glucose profile (as above).
- ☒ Treatment is indicated for glucose levels ≥ 5.8 mmol/L.
- ☒ Dietary control should be attempted initially. If this is not successful then insulin should be prescribed. Management is then as above for established diabetes.

Labour and delivery

- ☒ When diabetes is well controlled and pregnancy is uncomplicated vaginal delivery between 38 and 40 weeks should be anticipated.

  — During labour close control of blood glucose is achieved by a continuous infusion of soluble insulin (usually 50 units in 50 ml normal saline), and a separate infusion of 5% dextrose with KCl (10 mmol in 500 ml) added. The dextrose and KCl infusion should run at a constant rate (100 ml/h)

  — Regular blood glucose monitoring should be undertaken and the insulin infusion titrated to keep levels between 5 and 7 mmol/L

  — If a syntocinon infusion is necessary this should be made up using normal saline

  — Continuous electronic fetal monitoring is advised.

- ☒ If elective caesarean section is planned, careful control is necessary before, during and afterwards until the woman can eat and drink normally.

- ☒ If pre-term labour supervenes, B-sympathomimetics and steroids are best avoided but, if absolutely necessary, can be covered by appropriate insulin infusions.

- ☒ As post partum haemorrahage is likely it is important that the blood group is identified with two pints of blood cross-matched.

Postnatal care

☒ Insulin sensitivity increases immediately after delivery of the placenta. The required dose of insulin therefore falls quickly and careful monitoring is necessary. Hence withhold the insulin injection after delivery and re-establish after assessing the blood sugar.

☒ Hypoglycaemia is common in the neonate and must be treated promptly.

☒ Breast-feeding is to be encouraged.

Perinatal mortality among diabetic women is now approaching that for other pregnancies (once congenital malformations are excluded), in the best centres.

Other endocrine problems

Pituiltary

Prolactin secretion increases from the anterior pituitary throughout pregnancy in response to oestrogen stimulation. By term the concentration has increased ten- to twenty-fold. Basal concentrations fall rapidly after delivery but remain above the normal range in lactating women. Suckling induces a prompt release and levels rise five- to ten-fold. Its main role in pregnancy is trophic action on the breast. After delivery it initiates and maintains lactation, and prevents ovulation (a contraceptive function).

Prolactinoma

Expansion of a prolactinoma is unusual during pregnancy. Conservative management is usually appropriate.

☒ If being treated with bromocriptine—stop it as soon as pregnancy is diagnosed.

☒ Check visual fields at 6-week intervals.

☒ If severe headaches develop or visual fields become impaired, admit to hospital. If fetal maturity allows, deliver, probably by caesarean section. As oestrogen levels fall the prolactin level and volume of the prolactinoma will fall. If the fetus is too immature give bromocriptine 5 mg daily, doubling each day to 20 mg/day in divided doses or until side-effects prevent further increase.

☒ If visual fields continue to deteriorate add dexamethasone to reduce intracranial swelling, and deliver by caesarean section within 48 hours.

☒ Breast-feeding is not contraindicated in the presence of a prolactinoma.

Thyroid

The main physiological changes in pregnancy are:

☒ Renal clearance of iodide doubles in the first trimester and then remains stable. The result is a low plasma iodide. This is only significant when dietary iodine intake is inadequate, when goitre can develop

☒ The level of thyroid-binding proteins (globulin, pre-albumin and albumin) more than doubles due to an oestrogen effect on the liver. Although total T3 and T4 levels rise markedly, the levels of free hormones fall gradually (but remain within normal limits) as pregnancy progresses

☒ Basal metabolic rate (BMR) increases by up to 30% by the third trimester. This is necessary because of the requirements of the uterus and fetus (75% of the change) and increased maternal respiratory and cardiac effort (25% of the change)

☒ Thyroid-stimulating hormone (TSH) levels are unchanged in pregnancy

☒ The pregnant woman is basically euthyroid.

Hyperthyroidism

☒ Complicates 2/1000 pregnancies but has usually been diagnosed and treated before pregnancy.

☒ The main cause is Graves' disease, but toxic multinodular or solitary nodular goitre may occur. Solitary nodules require careful evaluation because of the risk of malignancy. Fine-needle aspiration is appropriate.

☒ Uncontrolled hyperthyroidism is associated with increased risk of IUGR, pre-term labour and fetal and neonatal death. The most frequent cause is an auto-antibody which crosses the placenta. It may cause neonatal hyperthyroidism, which has a high mortality rate (up to 25% of cases).

Signs and symptoms
The symptoms overlap with those of normal pregnancy, and palpable thyroid enlargement may be physiological in pregnancy. Biochemical diagnosis is essential.

Diagnosis Free T3 raised; free T4 raised or normal; TSH suppressed.

Treatment Carbimazole or propylthiouracil with thyroxine supplement.

- ☒ These drugs cross the placenta and can therefore affect the fetal thyroid. However, the balance of risk is in their favour. When control is achieved the drugs can be reduced gradually.

- ☒ Propranolol may be used to control serious peripheral effects of thyrotoxicosis.

- ☒ Breast-feeding is not necessarily contraindicated.

- ☒ Sub-total thyroidectomy may be indicated if a large goitre is causing obstruction, drugs fail to control the symptoms, or there -are toxic reactions to drugs.

- ☒ Babies born to thyrotoxic mothers should be screened for hypothyroidism.

Hypothyroidism

- ☒ The main causes of primary hypothyroidism are idiopathic, Hashimoto's thyroiditis and post-ablative.

- ☒ Treated hypothyroidism due to auto-immune disease or following partial thyroidectomy is not uncommon (about 9/1000 pregnancies).

- ☒ Untreated hypothyroidism in early pregnancy has a high fetal wastage or can lead to mental retardation, deafness and cerebral palsy. Later in pregnancy cretinism results.

- ☒ Myxoedema rarely presents in pregnancy because sufferers tend to be infertile.

Signs and symptoms

Cold intolerance, changes in skin or hair texture, delayed reflexes, bradycardia. A goitre may be present.

Diagnosis

Free T4 reduced; TSH high. These can also be used to lost adequacy of replacement therapy.

Treatment Thyroxine replacement.

- ☒ Breast-feeding is not contraindicated.

- ☒ If mother has previously had thyrotoxicosis, check for neonatal thyrotoxicosis. If she has had auto-immune thyroiditis, check baby for hypothyroidism.

Postpartum thyroiditis

- This is said to occur in 5-9% of pregnancies and is generally unrecognised.

- It presents with fatigue, palpitations or other features of mild hyperthyroidism 2-4 months postpartum, and is often confused with 'postpartum blues'.

- It is commonly associated with HLA DR3, 4 or 5.

- Up to 25% of affected women will have a first-degree relative with a history of thyroid disease. Such women should be screened for thyroid antibodies at booking.

Diagnosis T3 and T4 levels are raised. Radioactive iodine uptake is low. Thyroid antimicrosomal antibodies are present.

Treatment Postpartum thyroiditis is usually a self-limiting condition, but hypothyroidism may persist in a small minority. In the thyrotoxic phase (3-blocking agents may be used: In the hypothyroid phase thyroxine can be given for 4-6 months.

Adrenal cortex

Among the physiological changes which occur in pregnancy are:
- Aldosterone levels rise within days of conception due to an increase in angiotensin II. This reaction is necessary in pregnancy to conserve sodium

- Plasma cortisol levels, both bound and free, are elevated with loss of the normal diurnal variation. This increase is due to a slight rise in ACTH as a result of placental secretion

- Deoxycorticosterone (DOC) shows the largest increase of all adrenal steroids, starting by 8 weeks' gestation. DOC is not suppressible by dexamethasone during pregnancy. It may be intimately involved with parturition

- Plasma testosterone rises secondary to the rise in sex hormone-binding globulin, although it is likely that unbound testosterone is unchanged.

Cushing's syndrome

- ☒ This is a rare but serious condition in pregnancy.

- ☒ Fetal loss is common and there is a significant risk to the mother's life.

- ☒ The main causes are pituitary adenoma, and adrenocortical adenoma or carcinoma.

- ☒ The presentation is as in the non-pregnant.

Adrenal medulla—Phaeochromocytoma

- ☒ The catecholamines adrenaline and noradrenaline do not change in pregnancy.

- ☒ This tumour rarely complicates pregnancy, but the consequences for the mother are serious if it goes undetected. Only about half the cases are diagnosed antenatally.

- ☒ Patients may present with sustained or paroxysmal hypertension. The other classical symptoms of headache, palpitations and excess sweating may not occur in pregnancy.

- ☒ It can cause sudden collapse in pregnancy, labour or the puerperium.

- ☒ It should be excluded:

- — when severe or intermittent hypertension occurs (particularly in early pregnancy)

    - — in the presence of above 'classical' symptoms

    - — in women with a family history of phaeochromocytoma or associated syndromes, e.g. neurofibromatosis or multiple endocrine neoplasia.

Diagnosis Estimation of catecholamines in a properly collected 24-hour urine sample. Ultrasound may detect a suprarenal mass. CT ,&/ or MRI are useful for further localisation.

Treatment α-adrenergic blockade using phenoxybenzamine.
- ☒ Control may take 10-14 days.

- ☒ Beta adrenergic blockade using propanolol may be necessary to treat tachyarrhythmias. cc-blockade must be achieved first.

- ☒ Before 23 weeks' gestation the tumour should be removed. From 24 weeks' gestation the pregnant uterus makes this technically difficult. Surgical removal can be delayed until fetal maturity is adequate as long as cc-blockade is achieved.

⊠ Removal should be considered with elective caesarean section. Specialist anaesthesia is required, and initial postoperative management must be in an intensive care unit.

Immunological disorders

For a description of the immune system and its function see Further Reading. The major factors protecting the semi-allogeneic (foreign) fetus and placenta from maternal immune attack are:

⊠ The absence of class I (HLA A,B,C) and class II (HLA DR DQ, DR) major histocompatibility complex (MHC) antigens from villous trophoblast

⊠ The presence on extravillous trophoblast of non-classical MHC antigens to which T cells cannot respond

⊠ Protective responses may occur to minor trophoblast antigens

⊠ Local immune response may be suppressed by non-specific suppressor cells and other factors in the maternal decidua.

The placenta acts as a barrier to the passage of maternal cells to the fetus. IgG, but not IgM, is actively transported. This provides passive immunity to the fetus but can also cause pathology, e.g. Rhesus haemolytic disease, and allo-immune thrombocytopenia.

Immune thrombocytopenia

Platelet mass and turnover increase in pregnancy. The count may fall slightly in normal pregnancy. Thrombocytopenia is defined as a platelet count below $100 \times 10^9 L^{-1}$ but major clinical concern arises at counts around $50 \times 10^9 L^{-1}$. **Auto-immune (or idiopathic) thrombocytopenia (ITP)** Affects about 1/1000 pregnancies.

⊠ IgG antiplatelet auto-antibodies bind to platelet-specific antigens and cause them to be sequestered in the spleen.

⊠ ITP occurs more commonly in women than in men, with a peak incidence at the height of the reproductive years.

Maternal risks have been overstated. The major hazard is postpartum haemorrhage with an incidence of over 30% if platelet count is below $100 \times 10^9 L^{-1}$.
Fetal risk

⊠ The IgG antiplatelet antibodies cross the placenta, but maternal platelet count is a poor predictor of fetal/neonatal thrombocytopenia.

- The principal fetal risk is intracranial haemorrhage (ICH) but this has been overstated.

- There is no evidence that elective caesarean section reduces the risk, but it is indicated in the pre-term infant and for breech presentation. However forceps and vacuum are unsuitable.

Investigation of mother with ITP

- If platelet count $\geq 100 \times 10^9 L^{-1}$ check it at booking, 28 and 34 weeks, and at onset of labour.

- If count $<50 \times 10^9 L^{-1}$, or if there is haemorrhage, exclude other causes —e.g. clotting disorder, pre-eclampsia. The value of measuring platelet auto-antibodies is not proven.

Investigation of fetus

- Antenatal ultrasound can help to exclude ICH in utero.

- Fetal scalp sampling in labour is not helpful.

- Cordocentesis will give an accurate picture of the fetal state but its morbidity does not justify its use except under exceptional circumstances.

Treatment

- *Corticosteroids*—if maternal platelet count $<50 \times 10^9 L^{-1}$.

- *Immunoglobulin infusion* is best restricted to steroid-resistant cases.

- *Platelet transfusions* give only short-lived benefit. They can be used to cover delivery if platelet count is $<30 \times 10^9 L^{-1}$.

- *Plasmaphoresis* may be used when other medical management has failed.

- Any woman who has had a splenectomy should take daily oral penicillin for life to protect against pneumococcal infections. A normal platelet count in a woman who has had a splenectomy does not mean that the fetus will be unaffected.

Feto-maternal allo-immune thrombocytopenia (FMAITP)

FMAITP is analogous to Rhesus disease.

- The incidence may be as high as 1-2/1000 pregnancies.

- The majority of cases in a Caucasian population are due to antibodies against the platelet antigens HPA-1a (75%) or HPA-5b (20%). The remainder are due to antibodies against other antigens (HPA-1 to HPA-9).

- Maternal platelets are normal but the fetus is at significant risk of intracranial haemorrhage.

- I lie first pregnancy is affected in up to 50% of cases, as are almost 100% of subsequent pregnancies in which the fetus is antigen-positive.

- Routine screening for maternal anti-platelet antibodies during pregnancy is currently only at the trial stage.

- II FMAITP is suspected or has been confirmed in a previous pregnancy:

    — check maternal serum for anti-platelet antibodies

    — determine maternal and paternal HPA status if not already known.

- Fetal HPA status can be ascertained by cell culture from amniocentesis or from fetal lymphocytes or platelets obtained by cordocentesis.

- The fetal platelet count can also be determined by cordocentesis and fetal immunoglobulin or platelets can be given if required.

- Elective caesarean section is indicated if the fetal platelet count is; <50 $\times 10^9 L^{-1}$.

Feto-maternal allo-immune neutropenia (FAN)

- This is the neutrophil equivalent of FMAITP which also can affect first pregnancies.

- The incidence is 0.5-1/1000 livebirths.

- Its clinical significance relates to the infant's ability to combat infection.

- Investigation is as above. Cordocentesis is more difficult to justify because of the less favourable fetal risk/benefit ratio as compared to FMAITP.

Systemic lupus erythematosus (SLE)

A multisystem disease of unknown aetiology that tends to occur in women of reproductive age.

☒ The diagnosis rests on the presence of criteria suggested by the American Rheumatism Association. The most helpful serological tests are anti-nuclear factor and anti-DNA antibodies.

☒ Pregnancy has no specific effects on SLE except for an increased risk of exacerbation during the puerperium.

☒ Women with SLE in pregnancy have an increased risk of:

- — first-trimester pregnancy loss
- — lupus nephritis
- — hypertension in pregnancy
- — transient neonatal SLE—permanent congenital heart block may occur in association with anti-Ro antibodies.

☒ A seemingly healthy woman delivering a baby with CHB should be observed for the development of SLE.

Management during pregnancy

☒ Close antenatal supervision is necessary, with particular attention to serial measurements of blood pressure, renal function and fetal growth.

☒ The mainstay of treatment is maternal corticosteroid therapy but azathioprine may be needed in some circumstances.

☒ The timing of delivery depends on the severity of the condition, and deteriorating renal function may be an indication for early delivery.

☒ If the fetus has congenital heart block then caesarean section is warranted.

Lupus anticoagulant (LA) or inhibitor is a circulating anticardiolipin antibody which acts on the clotting cascade.

☒ All phospholipid-dependent coagulation tests, e.g. activated partial thromboplastin time (APTT) and kaolin clotting time (KCT), tend to be prolonged even after the addition of normal plasma.

☒ It is associated with a high prevalence of maternal thrombosis and fetal loss.

- ☒ It is not specific to SLE and may be found in any woman with a history of unexplained fetal loss at any gestational age.

- ☒ Corticosteroids and low-dose aspirin have been used successfully to treat affected women.

Myasthenia gravis

A rare auto-immune condition with a peak incidence between 20 and 30 years of age frequently associated with a thymoma or thymic lymphoid hyperplasia.
- ☒ It produces rapid fatigue and weakness of voluntary muscles.

- ☒ Pregnancy does not worsen the disease but exacerbations can occur (most frequently in the puerperium) in up to 30% of women.

- ☒ The antibody can cross the placenta and cause a transient (or rarely permanent) effect on fetal voluntary muscles.

- ☒ Among the drugs which can exacerbate it are sedatives, tranquillisers, analgesics and narcotics.

- ☒ Treatment is with anticholinesterase drugs such as neostigmine (with atropine) or pyridostigmine. Corticosteroids or ACTH may also be effective.

- ☒ Labour may be shorter than usual but the effort of the second stage can be tiring. Elective forceps delivery is usually indicated.

- ☒ General anaesthesia requiring muscle relaxation can result in prolonged paralysis of voluntary muscles.

Rhesus iso-immunisation the RH factor

- ☒ The Rh gene is made up of three components from three allelomorphic pairs—C or D or d, E or e. Each parent passes on either the first or second half of his/her full genotype, e.g. CDe/cde parents hand on their CDe or cde.

- ☒ All Rh-negative people have'd' in each half of the genotype. Where 'D' occurs in both halves of the genotype a parent is homozygous and passes on only the Rh-D-positive gene.

- ☒ Clinically significant rhesus iso-immunisation is usually against the D antigen. Anti-c or anti-Kell antibodies may also cause problems.

Sensitisation

☒ Sensitisation may occur antenatally in 1-2% of previously unsensitised Rh-D-negative women in the absence of any overt complications.

☒ It usually occurs at parturition due to feto-maternal haemorrhage.

☒ Other causes of transplacental haemorrhage include abortion (spontaneous or induced), abruptio placentae, amniocentesis and external cephalic version.

Prevention

☒ Anti-D immunoglobulin 500 i.u. (100 lag) can eliminate up to 4.0 ml of Rh-D-positive blood from the maternal circulation.

☒ It should be given in this dose to all Rh-D-negative women within 60 hours of delivering a Rh-D-positive infant from 20 weeks' gestation (or after a severe placental abruption). If a Kleihauer test demonstrates a feto-maternal transfusion (FMT) of >4.0 ml, additional anti-D must be given.

☒ 250 i.u. (50 ug) should be given to Rh-D-negative women as soon as possible after a potentially sensitising event. Any FMT >2.0 ml requires additional anti-D.

☒ Anti-D 500 i.u. at 28 and 34 weeks should be given to Rh-Dnegative primigravidae and other previously unsensitised women. This would reduce the incidence of Rh sensitisation by at least a factor of 8.

☒ The continued occurrence of Rh iso-immunisation is due to failure to give any or enough anti-D when indicated.

Detection

In unsensitised women check for Rh antibodies at booking, 28, 32 and 36 weeks.

Prediction of severity

Obstetric history

☒ It tends to become more severe in successive pregnancies.

☒ If at least one child has died from Rhesus haemolytic disease the chance of this pregnancy ending successfully is less than 50%.

Paternal genotype

☒ About 75% of the fathers of affected children are homozygous (R1R1)

Maternal antibody levels

☒ Once antibodies are detected they must be measured at least monthly thereafter.

☒ Serum antibody protein levels are of greater predictive value than antibody titres.

☒ A rapid increase suggests that acute haemolysis will be occurring in the fetus, and amniotic fluid analysis is necessary.

Amniotic fluid analysis
☒ Maternal IgG crosses the placenta and will cause a fetal haemolytic anaemia.

☒ If a previous pregnancy has been complicated by Rhiso-immunisation, the first amniocentesis should be 10 weeks before the earliest previous intrauterine transfusion, intrauterine death or delivery of a fatally or severely affected infant, but not before 20 weeks' gestation.

☒ The second should be 3-4 weeks later. The necessity for, and interval between, subsequent amniocenteses are determined by bilirubin levels.

Fetal blood sampling
☒ Fetal blood sampling under ultrasound guidance can be used to check fetal haematocrit.

☒ It is indicated in patients at risk of severe early disease as indicated by hyperdynamic middle cerebral artery Doppler velocities. Peak systolic velocity (PSV) of more than 50ml/s indicates a hyperdynamic status.

Intrauterine transfusion
☒ If the fetus is severely affected between 24 and 31 weeks' gestation, direct intravascular fetal blood transfusion (IVT) can be carried out under ultrasound guidance; transfusions can be repeated fortnightly.

☒ It is particularly useful if hydrops is present, but should be carried out only in specialised centres.

☒ Intraperitoneal transfusion can be used in conjunction with IVT in the absence of hydrops.

Testing the baby at birth
Cord blood is taken routinely from the babies of all Rh-D-negative mothers for Hb and film, Direct/Indirect Coombs' test and serum bilirubin levels.

Respiratory disease

Bronchial asthma

- ☒ Pregnancy has no consistent effect on asthma, and cases should be managed medically in the normal manner using sympathomimetic bronchodilators (e.g. salbutamol or orciprenaline) or disodium cromoglycate.

- ☒ If steroids are used, or have been recently, cover labour (for anaesthesia) with hydrocortisone (inhaled steroids do not need parenteral cover during labour).

- ☒ Status asthmaticus is treated by steroids in high doses, bronchodilators and artificial ventilation, if necessary.

Pulmonary tuberculosis

- ☒ If the diagnosis is made during pregnancy, treat with the standard regimen. (pyrazinamide for 2 months and isoniazid with rifampicin for 6 months. Pyridoxine supplements are advised. Do not use streptomycin in pregnancy.

- ☒ Breast-feeding is contrainclicatecl if the patient has sputum-positive TB.

- ☒ The infant requires BCG vaccination and should be separated from the mother only if she has open TB and until Mantoux conversion.

Epilepsy

- ☒ Pre-pregnancy counselling is important for women with epilepsy in order to:

  — check their anticonvulsant therapy for need, safety and dosage

  — allay their many fears about pregnancy and nursing a small baby.

- ☒ Pregnancy does not provoke epilepsy in mothers but the frequency of seizures may increase because anticonvulsants are cleared more quickly.

- ☒ The risk of an epileptic mother having an epileptic baby is about 1/40.

Teratogenecity of anticonvulsants

- ☒ The incidence of congenital malformations is increased two- to three-fold in infants of women on anticonvulsants.

☒ No one drug is free of risk, but phenytoin (alone or in combination) is implicated most frequently.

☒ Among the problems are:

— cleft lip and/or palate (increased ten-fold)

— congenital heart defect (increased four-fold)

— hypoplasia of terminal phalanges of fingers

— possible characteristic facial appearance: wide-spaced eyes, low posterior hair line, short neck, prominent brow and trigoncephaly

— retarded growth, delayed development and, occasionally, mental retardation.

☒ Sodium valproate is associated with fetal spina bifida in about 1% of 'at risk' pregnancies.

Management

☒ Prescribe anticonvulsants in doses sufficient to prevent convulsions.

☒ Single-drug therapy should be aimed for if possible.

☒ Vitamin K should be given to all neonates (1 mg i.m.).

☒ Breast-feeding is not contraindicated.

☒ Status epilepticus is best treated with intravenous diazepam. The airway must be kept patent and oxygen administered.

Incidence approximately 1/1500 pregnancies.

Jaundice caused by pregnancy

Intrahepatic cholestasis (20% of cases)

☒ The patient has pruritus in the second half of pregnancy (some never become jaundiced).

☒ Bilirubin and transaminases are slightly elevated.

☒ It is associated with some increased risk of pre-term labour, fetal distress and perinatal death.

☒ It clears up after delivery and does not proceed to chronic liver disease.

- ☒ It tends to recur in subsequent pregnancies and may also occur in association with oestrogen-containing oral contraceptives.

- ☒ Cholestyramine/ Udehep will reduce itching but is very unpleasant to take. Parenteral vitamin K is required if jaundice causes prolongation of the prothrombin time.

Jaundice complicating pre-eclampsia

Intercurrent jaundice in pregnancy

Viral hepatitis (40% of cases)

Due either to hepatitis B or C (long incubation, serum hepatitis) or hepatitis A (short incubation, infective hepatitis). Hepatitis B is discussed on page 109.

Cholelithiasis (6% of cases)
- ☒ Modern ultrasound or transhepatic cholangiography may be useful in confirming the diagnosis.

- ☒ Cholecystectomy can be carried out in pregnancy if necessary, preferably not earlier or later than the second trimester.

Drug toxicity and haemolysis
These are rare causes, but should be considered.

Pre-existing liver disease
- ☒ Pregnancy is uncommon in the presence of cirrhosis due, for example, to active chronic hepatitis, or primary biliary cirrhosis.

- ☒ The prognosis is good for mother and baby in familial non-haemolytic jaundice, e.g. Gilbert's and the Dubin-Johnson syndromes. Pregnancy may increase jaundice in the latter.

Gastric reflux and hiatus hernia

The lower oesophageal sphincter relaxes under the influence of pregnancy hormones. Reflux of acid gastric contents leads to heartburn. This can also be due to a 'sliding' hiatus hernia.
Management
- ☒ Frequent small meals; advise patient to avoid lying flat; simple antacids.

- ☒ If no relief is obtained, 'floating' antacids, or metoclopramide, can be tried.

Coeliac disease

- ☒ Coeliac disease may present in pregnancy as a folate deficiency anaemia.

- ☒ If untreated it may be associated with an increased risk of abortion or IUGR.

- ☒ It is successfully treated by a gluten-free diet and vitamin supplements.

Ulcerative colitis

- ☒ Ulcerative colitis does not affect pregnancy adversely.

- ☒ Pregnancy does not increase the chance of relapse of quiescent colitis, but if the colitis arises de novo in pregnancy or the puerperium it carries a poor prognosis.

- ☒ Treatment can continue during pregnancy with rectal and systemic steroids and/or sulphasalazine.

- ☒ In the presence of an ileostomy most pregnancies proceed to normal vaginal delivery.

Crohn's disease

- ☒ There may be a small adverse effect on fetal outcome due to the disease.

- ☒ The condition itself is usually unaffected by pregnancy.

- ☒ Deterioration is most likely in the puerperium.

- ☒ It should be managed in the same manner as in the nonpregnant.

Phsychiatric disorders

Postpartum 'blues'
- ☒ This is not an illness but rather a transient mild disturbance characterised by:

— weeping

— irritability

— variation in mood
— feelings of helplessness

— sensitivity to criticism

— poor sleep.

- ☒ It occurs in at least 50% of postpartum women, usually develops around the third day, and may last for a few hours or days.
- ☒ Treatment is by psychological support and reassurance.

Depressive illness

- ☒ This is characterised by tiredness, lethargy, irritability and anxiety, which may be more prominent than depression.
- ☒ It is often brought on by psycho-social stress, and there may be a previous psychiatric history.
- ☒ Its peak incidence is 3 months postpartum.
- ☒ Treatment is by psychological and practical support and antidepressant drugs as necessary.

Puerperal psychosis

- ☒ The incidence is about 2/1000 live births.
- ☒ Puerperal psychosis presents either as an affective disorder with depression or hypomania, or schizophrenia with delusions and hallucinations.
- ☒ It often begins within 4 days of delivery.
- ☒ A psychiatrist must be consulted because there is risk of suicide and harm to or neglect of the baby.
- ☒ There is an increased risk of psychotic illness in the future, including during further pregnancies.
- ☒ Monoamine oxidase inhibitors are best avoided in pregnancy, but withdrawal must be gradual.

Thrombosis and thromboembolism
Coagulation and fibrinolysis during normal prgnancy

- ☒ Factors VII, VIII, IX and X are increased from the beginning of the second trimester. The most marked increase is in plasma fibrinogen. This results in a relative hypercoagulable state ready to cope with placental separation at delivery.

- ☒ Plasma fibrinolytic activity is decreased because plasmin inhibitors (e.g. a 2- macroglobulin and a,-antitrypsin) increase substantially.

- ☒ Fibrinolysis returns to normal within 15 minutes of delivery of the placenta.

- ☒ These were the commonest causes of maternal death in the developed countries from 1991-93, making up over 25% of the total.

- ☒ Of the 35 deaths, 30 were from pulmonary thromboembolism (PTE) and five from cerebral thrombosis. Another five deaths from PTE occurred beyond the 42nd day.

- ☒ In the deaths from PTE, 12 occurred antepartum, one intrapartum and 17 postpartum.

- ☒ Of the 17 postpartum PTE deaths, 13 (76%) followed caesarean section, as did all five from cerebral thrombosis.

Factors associated with increased risk
☒ Mild risk factors

- — requires early mobilisation and hydration:

- — elective caesarean section in an uncomplicated pregnancy with no other risk markers

- — blood groups other than O.

☒ Moderate risk factors
- — consider prophylaxis

- — maternal age >35 years. The risk in women aged over 40 years is 60 times that for those aged 25 or less

- — parity 4 or more

- — obesity (>80 kg) associated with poor mobility and venous stasis

- — gross varicose veins

- — proteinuric pre-eclampsia

- — any surgical procedure in labour (particularly emergency caesarean section)

- — immobility before surgery (>4 days)

- — sickle cell disease, major intercurrent illness or infection.

☒ **High risk factors**—requires heparin and leg stockings: — three or more moderate risk factors

- personal or family history of thrombosis. The risk of recurrence in a woman with a past history of thromboembolism occurring in pregnancy or while on 'the pill' is-about 12%, the majority of which are postnatal

- 'thrombophilia', i.e. antithrombin III, protein C or protein S deficiencies; activated protein C resistance (due to the presence of factor V Leiden), MTHFR Mutation

- anti-cardiolipin syndrome or presence of lupus inhibitor

- major surgery, e.g. caesarean hysterectomy.

Incidence

☒ The incidence of non-fatal TE in pregnancy is not known.

☒ Deep vein thrombosis (DVT) complicates about 2% of caesarean sections.

Deep vein thrombosis

☒ The most common clinical features are pain, local tenderness, swelling, oedema, a positive Homan's sign, a change in leg colour and temperature and a palpable thrombosed vein.

☒ Most cases are less obvious and some are silent. Clinical diagnosis is therefore unreliable.

☒ Over 80% are left-sided.

☒ (Superficial thrombophlebitis does not carry a significant risk of thromboembolism unless it extends to the deep veins.)

Diagnosis

☒ Venography is the 'gold standard'.

☒ Ultrasonic detection of venous patency is inadequate.

☒ Radioactive fibrinogen uptake is contraindicated.

The main complications are pulmonary embolism and chronic vascular insufficiency.

Pulmonary embolism

There may be no prior clinical evidence of DVT.
Signs and symptoms: Pleuritic pain, haemoptysis, dyspnoea and varying degrees of shock. Consider also if there is no other obvious explanation for tachycardia, pyrexia or bronchospasm.
Investigation

☒ Chest X-ray may be helpful but can be totally normal.

☒ ECG—usually normal except when the embolus is large and has produced acute cor pulmonale. Even these changes may be obscured by the usual ECG changes which occur in pregnancy.

☒ Ventilation-perfusion isotope (VQ) lung scan.

☒ Pulmonary angiography may need to be considered.

Management of DVT and pulmonary embolism

Heparin does not cross the placenta or reach breast milk so there is no added risk to the fetus. Its action is to inhibit thrombin and factors IX, X, XI and XII.

☒ Acute therapy—intravenous calcium heparin 40 000 units daily (in saline by infusion pump) for at least 48 hours.

☒ Long-term therapy—subcutaneous heparin inhibits activated factor X without prolonging the clotting time. Use a twice-daily unfractionated heparin or a single daily dose of low molecular weight heparin. This does not add to the risk of haemorrhage even at caesarean section. Continue for at least 6 weeks postpartum (or warfarin may be substituted after delivery).

☒ Side-effects of long-term therapy include allergic reactions, thrombocytopenia and maternal osteopenia, which is dose- and duration-dependent with some unpredictable individual susceptibility.

Warfarin inhibits the synthesis of vitamin K-dependent clotting factors (II, VII, IX and X). It crosses the placenta readily but not significantly in breast milk.

☒ It is best avoided in the first trimester because of a slight risk of embryopathy.

☒ Even with meticulous control (prothrombin time 2-2.5 times the clotting time for a normal control plasma), there is an increased risk of fetal haemorrhage.

☒ Its anticoagulant effect cannot be reversed rapidly.

treat women with history of TE who are admitted to hospital for bed rest).

- ☒ **Regional anaesthesia?**—epidural or spinal block is contraindicated if patient is fully anticoagulated. However, there is no evidence that prophylactic heparin increases the risk of spinal haematoma. Each case must be judged on its merits.

Malignant disease and pregnancy

Pregnancy does not usually adversely affect the course of malignant disease. The poor prognosis of pregnant women with cervical cancer is more likely to be due to the aggressiveness of the tumour in women in that age group than to the pregnancy itself.

Cervical cancer and cervical intraepithelial neoplasia

- ☒ Offer a cervical smear at the booking antenatal clinic if the women has never had one before or not within the past 5 years.

- ☒ If the smear is abnormal carry out colposcopy (colposcopically directed biopsies can be taken safely in pregnancy).

Cervical intraepithelial neoplasia (CIN) should be serially observed for the remainder of pregnancy and dealt with definitively at the end of the puerperium.

Invasive carcinoma of the cervix

Fite condition poses several clinical problems in pregnancy.

- ☒ If discovered under 22 weeks' gestation advise termination (by hysterotomy) followed by definitive treatment.

- ☒ Between 22 and 26 weeks it may be justifiable to await fetal viability before ending the pregnancy.

- ☒ Thereafter, delivery should be effected in consultation with a neonatal paediatrician and the woman herself.

- ☒ Vaginal delivery is contraindicated.

Whatever the management, the prognosis is poor.

Ovarian cancer

- ☒ Ovarian tumors of all varieties are said to complicate 1/1000 pregnancies, although only 1 in 20 are malignant. The frequency of tumor types is as in the non-pregnant woman.

☒ Ultrasound is useful for detection of ovarian swellings.

Management
☒ Treat as in the non-pregnant woman.

☒ The prognosis seems to be better for ovarian cancer in pregnancy, with a 5-year survival rate of up to 75% compared to an overall 25%. This reflects the nature of the tumors in this age group.

Breast cancer
☒ This is the commonest malignant tumour to affect women. About 2% of women under 45 years of age who have the disease are pregnant at the time of diagnosis.

☒ Lymph node involvement seems to be increased in pregnancy. Prognosis may therefore be poorer.

Management
☒ In the first half of pregnancy, treatment should be as for the non-pregnant woman; if chemotherapy is necessary,therefore termination is recommended.

☒ In the second half of pregnancy, if the pregnancy is close to viability there may be an option of extending the pregnancy upto 30-32 weeks so a live fetus can be delivered. Immediately following the delivery patient is referred for definitive management, however in general cancer surgeries of any descipline during the puerpariam carries high risk of mortality and morbidity attributed to venus thrombosis, haemorrhage, sepsis and breakdown of the tissues/anastomoses.

☒ Breast-feeding is probably contraindicated, especially if the women is on chemotherapy

☒ Further pregnancies can be embarked on if desired after a post treatment interval of at least 2 years.

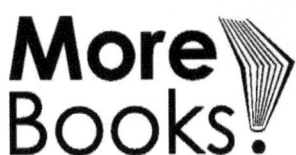
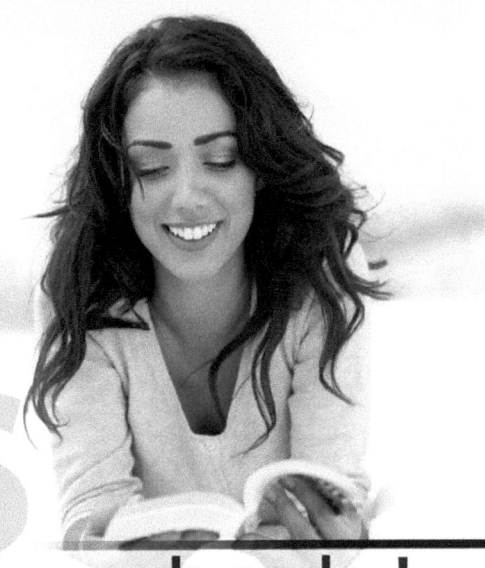
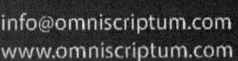
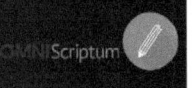

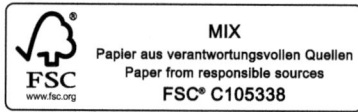